I0789335

Energetics CrossTherapy

Healing Techniques and Trances
Volume 1

Christophe Pank

Table des matières

Author of :

1/ My first steps on the Law of Attraction (Feb 2013)

2/ Journey of a Hypnosis practitioner against cancer (Fev 2015)

3/ Hypnosis and Pain Management : The study of the Hypno-Analgesia Process (Jul 2015)

4/ Limited Power : Accepting our own limits is to open up our real potential (May 2016)

5/ Hyperempiria and Self-Mastery : Apply Hyperempiria for your personal development (Jul 2017)

Introduction

Since I started to be so passionate about personal care and personal development, I always liked the energetic aspect. Martial arts are mainly the reason of this.

It is so easy to destroy, and so delicate to build, to heal. While I was learning to hit, to fight or even to beat, a part of myself got really interested in internal works. The 'internal' world in combat sport represents disciplines which work on the energy of the body : Ki/Chi or Prana.

This energy is not recognised by our scientific community, even if more and more admitted especially in acupuncture principles. As many practitioners of external works would recognise the complexity of the internal has been hard to admit. Moreover, I only believe what I live, so words in a book are not enough. Another way would have been to practice for 30 years to discover the results...but that is just a little too long for me. I can be impatient.

One day, I was participating in a Yi Chuan class and I was fortunate enough to see a Chinese teacher appease the twisted ankle of another practitioner...by laying hands only. It was a **revelation**. To not use the energy to destroy but to protect and heal.

So I started to lay hands...on me. Pains, physical hurts and step by step psychic ones, started to be erased only to leave behind well being. Honestly, it wasn't heaven aswell.

I was still quite stressed before a fight, still some fears that won't go and some hurts were really taking a long time to be appeased. However, everything seemed so 'logical'.

I was meditating, a mixture between zen and mostly indian meditations, **my hands 'were talking'**.

My body was living a lot of weird sensations. The more I was working on seated and standing meditations, as a tree, the more my being was awakening to **extraordinary things**. Today, I think that I was **opening myself to myself,** and yes, this is extraordinary. On my energetic path in many disciplines, I met many people who helped me to understand better, practice better and most of all, **gave me confidence** in what I was living. I think that **the most difficult is to 'believe'** what we feel, perceive despite our educated mind resisting it. On my path, I started to be aware, and **my subconscious too**, that these different phenomenon were put in place when **I was entering Trance**. A special moment where my conscious and subconscious **were in sync** to live together. The more I work on trances, the more I realise that we are capable of really surprising, positive and beneficial things and particularly in 'energetic care'.

In this book, I propose to you different techniques which you can **easily apply** without having to spend years of work, neither spend hundreds or even thousands of pounds/dollars in order to succeed. It is simple, accessible to all, and steps that you will go through will be personal. **I present a vision, not a truth,** a path, not THE path. Take what is useful for you whether you are a practitioner in energetics, therapy or a learner. Test it, make your own opinion, and if you like it, **share it**.

Chapter 1 : The Principle of Trance

Trance is a word which can be defined in many different ways. In Cross Therapy, I use a very simple definition : Phase of **communication between conscious and subconscious**, even with a part of the unconscious. *Trance is not an extraordinary phenomenon,* on the opposite it is a very common thing in our life. This communication is nearly permanent, it is just not necessarily *'useful'*. A day dream, an absence during a discussion, is a trance that we can have all day long.

Here is a lexicon, I would advise for you to keep in mind during your reading of this book, so that you can understand well what we are going to talk about.

- **Conscious :** Analytic part, logic of our personality, short term memory. Keep in mind that during trances, **conscious is always present.** It is also a way, for us, to understand some symbolic messages of our subconscious.

- **Subconscious :** Keeps all longterm memories and information since birth. Is the chair of our emotions and our capacity to find a way to be in the most 'optimum' state. This state is not necessarily the most pleasant, it is the 'less worst'.

- **Unconscious :** Handle our **physiological functioning** and our instinctive reactions to survive and live our daily life.

- **Critical Factor :** It is a transfer airlock which is divided into two parts.

1- The airlock **between the Conscious and Subconscious** permits us not to take all the information given as *suggestion-truth*. For example a child younger than 6 years old doesn't have any critical factor. Therefore, if you tell him that soda is water, with time, he will believe it and call soda, water. This airlock has a function to **filter information** in order to choose different options : refuse it and take it out / keep it in the airlock for 'réflection' / integrate it in the subconscious memory.

2- The airlock **between Subconscious and Conscious** prevents some things to come back to the conscious and create **an instability too strong** for *the homeostasis* of the being. Imagine that a trauma keeps coming back without being 'handled', it will cause a lot of disfunctions in the psyche, even in the body so that it becomes bearable. Besides, there is a belief which has been taught to me over time : '*We don't experience more than what we can handle*'. The more I study trances and psyche, the more I believe in this concept even if sometimes, **we wonder if it is possible to handle it all**.

Never in trances will the **critical factor** disappear, it is simply bypassed and can't play its initial role.
- **Trance :** *Communication between Conscious and Subconscious by bypassing the critical factor.* A trance doesn't have a unique form. Each trance we live will have a **different utility** and all will not be exploitable for our energetic or therapeutic objectives. During trances, there is a **more fluid dialogue** between the two parts of ourselves, without the barrier imposed by the critical factor.

As in all dialogue, it is possible that **one or the other expresses itself more.**
Indeed, sometimes subconscious will **be very present**, making us think that we are not in trance, but we are, there are disciplines which use well **this conscious trance** : the conversational hypnosis and the NLP. Let's take the example of a negotiation with the NLP tools. At no moment, either the interlocutor will close his eyes, or have the sensation to not be conscious of what he is doing or saying. However, these tools allow us to quickly validate the negotiation process.

Some other times, **subconscious will be omnipresent** and will only leave space to conscious *to understand* what is happening and then give it the necessary information. This is the reason why I often say that **trances are more or less stables.**

- **Stability of Trance :** Trances *are not in a frozen state.* Indeed with the different elements we talked about previously, we know that the **dialogue will vary** according to moments, emotions, desires, environment...In the same trance, we can live a moment **in full consciousness** of our hurts and gestures, then for a lapse of time only, listen to our instinct and feel that **our hands and words live by themselves**, becoming then an observer of this trance. The **critical factor will also make this state more unstable**, it suffices that one deep information comes back in the conscious to make a stop on it for the *trance which was deep, becomes more active.*

These different principles are important to understand, because they will be the base of our work in Energetics CT. The trance that we will live, will be **the door** to our perceptions, discoveries and energetic 'projections'. Meditations, magnetism sessions and extrasensory perceptions happen in trances for operators and the ones living the session : the partners.

Chapter 2 : How to go into Trances ?

From my point of view, whatever discipline we practice, **we all enter into trances** which allow us to **optimise** what we put in place, without talking about the world of better being, sport in particular. A runner enters into his trance as soon as he finds his rhythm, a tennis player doesn't pay any attention to what happens around him/her, his/her focus is on the ball. Swimming, with its work on respiration and our feedback is even more obvious…who ever left a pool without

a sensation of peace and serenity.

In energetic, it is as striking. You may be a magnetizer or a Reiki practitioner, you all have **your ways to focus back** before a session starts. This moment of **focusing on yourself is a trance.** Some use symbols, other mantras, other passages of a Holy book. The importance is to find back a state which permits you to offer a beautiful and positive strength.

In Energetic CT, I estimate that the **basic state** to reach is the trance. To do so, we are going to work on simple exercises which can lead to a trance.

Exercise 1 : Respiration

The first thing which can lead you into a trance is **your breathing**.

It is enough to remember of a moment where you were swimming to think back to how much you were in a **full relaxation state.**

Let's take a very easy exercise :

- Take your pulse at your wrist
- Inhale on 6 pulses
- Exhale on 6 pulses
- When you feel that you are relaxed and appeased, stop
- You are in a light trance.

Exercise 2 : Fix your eyes

When you talk to someone and you start day dreaming, you are still listening, however your eyes look in the emptiness. You are experiencing **a trance**.

Do this exercise :
- Take a point somewhere high
- Fix on this point with your eyes
- Really focus only on this point
- Notice all sounds around you, even silence
- Notice the sensations you live
- Keep your eyes fixed but now in a wider way
- Once you perceive all around you,
- Breathe deeply and keep this state

Exercise 3 : Act as If

Did you ever imagine yourself as somebody else ? Maybe in the morning, while preparing yourself ?

Or playing a role ? And it is perfect. This is an excellent means to bypass your critical factor.
Do this exercise :
- Act as if you were 5 years old
- Close your eyes
- After a few seconds, act as if your eyelids were glued
- Act as if you couldn't open them anymore
- Once your eyes are well relaxed, breathe 3 times deeply
- Open your eyes

Remember, trances are daily elements, it is a way to be more open with ourselves and these different rituals can help us. You can also make yourself your rituals :

- Music
- Incense
- Tai Chi
- Jump up and down
- Yell

...

Whatever works for you, what matters is to **put you in a different condition than your daily life,** it is in every energetic ritual. Indeed, traditional styles use **mantras, meditations or even prayers to enter into trance** which allow you to provide a session to a partner.
I would advise that you do at least once sophrology or hypnosis session so that you can qualify what is a trance and also create an anchor.

Chapter 3 : Cosmos Points

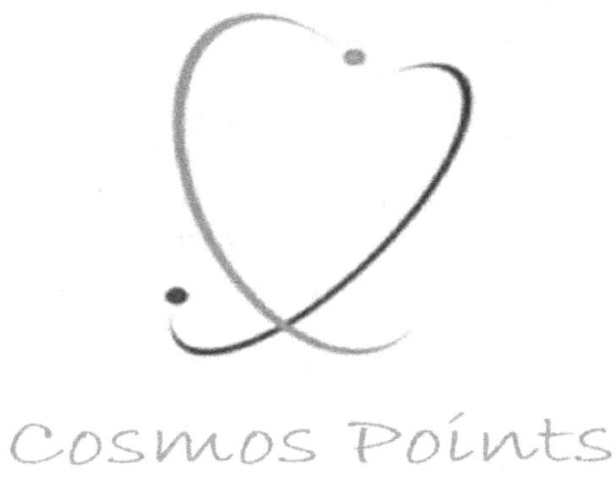

It is important that you have defined already your way to live trances.
Indeed, Cosmos Points are particular in their way to make us enter into a **subtle state of trance**, which opens up many capacities.

A – What is a Cosmos Point ?

It is a point linked to the **type of personalities** named Enneatype. It was **Alan Sheet** who was the first to talk about this under the name of 'Movement Centres'. He defined that respectively of the nine types of personality from the Enneagram, there are nine centres of energy.

In the limited information I was able to get, he defined them as **points to centre yourself**. It is important to note that Alan Sheet was a practitioner of Aikido.

A martial art, which has for goal the *union of energies'*.

When I understood that, to centre on these points, was allowing us to enter into a **balanced and harmonious trance**, I wondered how far we would be able to go. It is at this moment that I discovered that we could do quite extraordinary things. I put on my kimono and I went to figure out what these points had to offer. After a few different physical experiences which you can find here : www.points-cosmos.com (In French), here are the first conclusions I came to :

- Capacity to recover quicker
- Possibility to have some kind of 'protection' against punches, as old masters of martial arts.
- For example during martial arts demonstration, when we can't be uplifted from the ground, or pushed.
All of this available in **one instant**, thinking simply at the point which describes your personality. For me, this physical demonstration is very important as in the energetic world, everything is so intellectual and impalpable. Indeed, when we do an energetic session for a partner, we never really know **if it is a suggestion or if really something happens in other dimensions.**

Cosmos points have the capacity to **show us that physically, instantly, there is a change** which physiologically is very hard to explain. On the other hand, ancient indian or chinese culture explained very well these phenomenon through CHI or PRANA.

B – How to discover your Cosmos Point ?

There are two different ways to do it. The first one is the most interesting in my opinion.

Indeed, if you are studying this book, it is because you want to **work both on you and your partners.**

1) Study of yourself through the discovery of your Enneatype :
You can read different books about Enneagram, an advice that my teacher gave me at the beginning, **do not do any tests online.** I know that we all want to go fast, I am like this too, however in the quest of our personal development, it is good **to know when to take your time.**
To learn who we really are is a real progression and have the double benefit of opening trance and to make you discover facets of yourself.
Here I will go back to the 9 bases coming from the Pearl Approach
- Base 1 : Development Quest
- Base 2 : Approbation Quest
- Base 3 : Success Quest
- Base 4 : Authenticity Quest
- Base 5 : Knowledge Quest
- Base 6 : Security Quest
- Base 7 : Diversity and Novelty Quest
- Base 8 : Power Quest
- Base 9 : Tranquillity Quest

Look for which base you correspond to and you will have the number of your Cosmos Point.

After this, you just need to find it on the **Tiger Cosmos scheme (Artist : Mwana Pyro)**

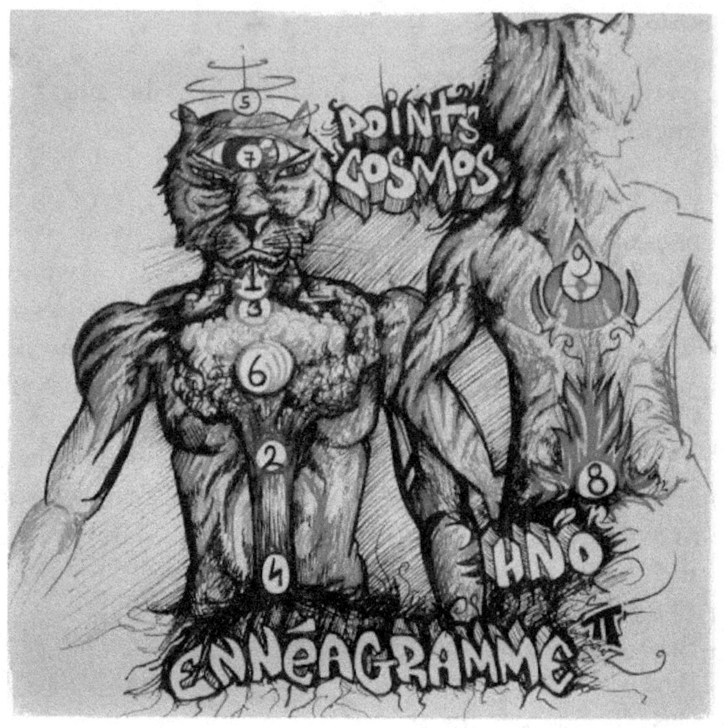

2) The second method is to **test directly all points :**
It is the quickest but not the most interesting for your development. I observed that very often a person who has **sensibilities, hurts or frequent pains** in a particular place, shows us the zone of his/her Cosmos Point.
For example, it happens often that those having a number 8 have pain in their lower back.

C – How to centre?

The basic centring

Before starting the tests, it is crucial to define **centre**.
 I received many mails on this subject. For many of us, who are used of complex techniques, to centre seems to be something asking an immense concentration.
In the case which concerns us, it is not a question of concentration. **It is a simple thought.** Yes, a simple thought, not more, not less.
To have tested the Cosmos Point in every possible direction, I realised that, the simple fact to just **think of the zone** of our Point is enough to have the results linked to it. Some have asked me if they should think of a very precise point. Except for the Point 1 and 3, all others can think of a zone.
With the experience, you will observe that the simple thought of this point, will 'activate' its presence, sometimes in a few seconds, sometimes a few minutes and after a while, for longer periods.

The advanced centring

The word 'advanced' here is pretentious as any learner can do this, it is only a way to dissociate the fact of thinking to the centre, and **'playing' with the centre.**
Indeed, you can , once the centring is operational put in place intentions. **The intention** is going to be a word, a sentence, a concept or an image that you will **inject into the centre.**

In other words, you are going to think of your centre **with one word,** for example : balance, relaxation.

D - Tests

Test 1 : The ring

The first one that you can do is the **ring.**
This test, I took it from an old book of *Sensei Koichi Tohei, in the book of Ki.*

Very simple, you can ask your partner to test you.
- Put your thumb and index finger in contact, keep the resistance.
- Your partner is going to make you open it, it will give you a reference to resistance.
- Now think of your Point (seen in your Enneatype), while keeping your thumb and index in contact.
- Your partner will try again to open your fingers.

Normally, if it is the right point, you are going to see that your partner **really struggles** to open them, even can't do it at all and you won't have the feeling that you need more strength.

This test needs to be approved by you. If you are not satisfied, just test another point. You are going to be surprised in how much one of the points is going to work better than any others.

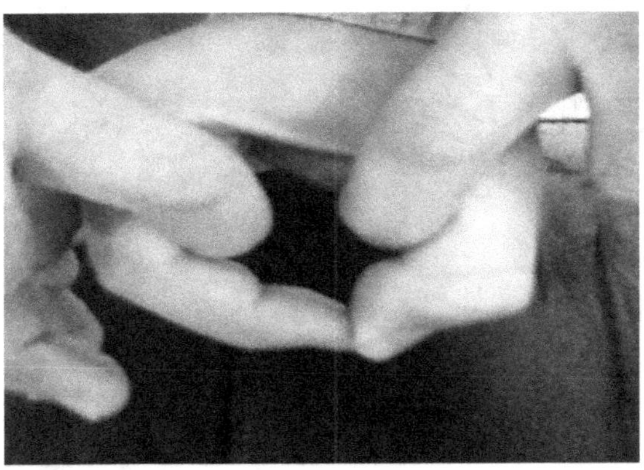

Test 2 : The Unflexible Arm

Just like the first test, try it out in order to gauge your natural resistance.

- Give your arm, the inside of the elbow up, and put it on the shoulder of your partner.
- His/her goal is to make you bend by pushing with his/her two hands on your elbow.
- Once you have your reference to resistance, try again.
- This time, centre yourself on your Cosmos Point and keep the resistance of your arm.

At this instant your arm will not bend and you don't have to put more strength into the action.

You do not need to do other tests, once this works, you can be sure of your Cosmos Point.

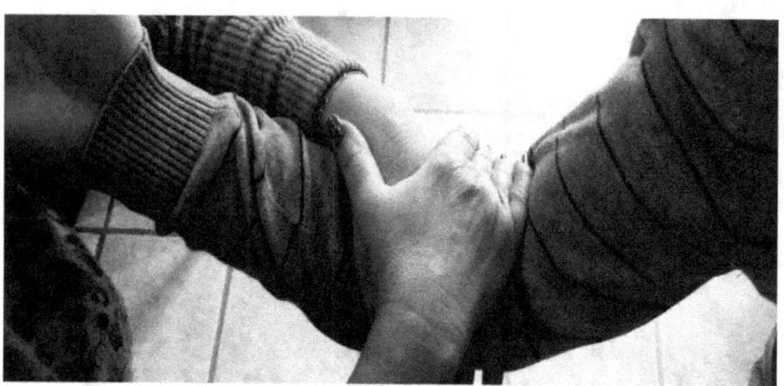

E – Encounter with these Cosmos Trances.

The amazing thing with the Cosmos Point is its **capacity to allow you to enter into a trance,** really positive and agreeable. Indeed, this centring brings us back to what is the most harmonious within us. This Trance permits us a first incursion in an internal well being. To learn how to use it correctly, I would advise that you centre *many times per day,* on your Cosmos Point.

Breathe calmy, think of this point and listen to yourself, to your body.

With this simple utilisation, you will be able to :

- Calm your insomnia
- Calm your anxiety
- Recover better from tiredness
- Handle better your stress
- Focus better

With only a few implications, you are going to be agreeably surprised by what this centre offers.

F – Cosmos Point and care on self

What I really like in these energetic technique processes, is the principle to **first work on yourself.** Too many therapists never use their techniques on themselves. They wait to be sick or very unwell to do what they should have done from the start.

I like the idea of chinese doctors who **teach us to never be sick.**

An energetic practitioner really has a great tool in his/her hands. And the **daily work** could be the key to the improvement of many things in his/her life. In this **Advanced Centring,** I was sharing to put *intentions* into the exercise. It is the starting point of your personal utilisation of the Cosmos Point.

- Centre yourself, until you *feel a better being*
- Put an **energetic intention** in your centre, you can imagine that you write it, put vitamins in it, jump up and down…anything. The thing is to link your action with the centre.
- Observe psychic and physiological changes.

If you are the type of person to **look for appeasement** in meditations or works in Qiqong :
- Centre yourself until you *feel a better being*
- Put your **quietude intention** in your centre, you can imagine Buddha in zazen, a peaceful chinese sifu.
- Observe psychic and physiological changes.
When you are in **pain,** sometimes, only to centre will take away the hurt. For others, it is better to follow this :
- Centre yourself until you *feel a better being*
- Put an **intention to completely suck up** the pain in your centre, you can imagine a vortex, a soothing light.
- Observe psychic and physiological changes.
For collecting hurts more than regularly following my trainings, this method is really efficient and easy to apply. You can do the same with the start of an illness like a cold. Practical applications are diverse. It is very easy to do, you just need to take a little bit of time and to experience. ,

G – Cosmos Point for the energetic share

As in magnetism, we can use Cosmos Point to **pass some energy** in order to calm down pains and appease people who ask for it. It is important that they do **ask for it**.
It is possible to develop the *saviour complex,* wishing to give away energy to everyone so that they feel better. However, if they didn't ask, I would advise not to.

You have now understood that the base of the work with Cosmos Point is **the centring and the intention.** When you want to work with someone, **you just need to lay your hands** on your partner.

- Hands in contact on your partner, wherever on the body, or directly on the pain.
- Centre yourself on your Cosmos Point
- Send an intention of appeasement to your partner. If you are more visual, you can imagine a healer, magnetizer…or otherwise.
- Repeat to yourself a word like : 'Appeasement', 'Unconditional Love', 'Happiness'…
- Ask how your partner feels regularly
When you do a session with someone else, propose a scale from 1 to 10 so that you know the discomfort level of your partner. You will then, easily support your partners.

H - Counter Argument

This title may seem a bit formal. I want to give you feedback on my own experiences with Cosmos Point. Don't be afraid, nothing really bad.

However, I still don't have any explanation for what follows.

Working on centring, I was interested in using it in the most optimum way. I had in mind to **continually centre.** Returns have been surprising. Indeed, as soon as we can **dissociate** what we do in our daily life and the part of us which stayed focused on the point, we can succeed to centre the majority of our day. Effects were not those expected. My body reacted very violently. I keep in mind though that *it may be that each Cosmos Point would give different results as would all the different personalities of the being.* During this period, I had very strong pain in my back, at certain times, I wouldn't feel my legs as I would permanently have pins and needles in my legs.

At the psychic level, from a state of agreeable at start, I went through intense and disturbing emotional variations. My body also started to put on weight without any particular reason. Let's resume this by saying that **at all levels, this period was excessive**. On the other hand, **I was in constant trance,** during which, I was **more sensitive** to all my different senses. My **intuitions were more precise** and during my sessions, I had really interesting connections with my clients. I maintained this experience for a few months, to be sure that I wasn't sabotaging myself…like a resistance that I would need to overcome. I was thinking that, as in energetics, a **cleaning period** was necessary. Well…even now I don't know. It was probably just too much at this time and by maturing my experience with the Cosmos Point and its use, I will maybe succeed to understand other things.

A little while after this experience, by playing with a tibetan bowl, I had the **beginning of an answer** on how to use this energy, this force. When you use a tibetan bowl, naturally, we want to become the master of the object.

We **impose our rhythm** to the vibration by turning faster and faster our hammer. Then the latter bounced, stopped the harmonic sound diffusing. **We break the energetic vibration of our action.** For the Cosmos Point, it is a bit the same. By centring continually **I wished to impose** my will to an energy which is, by nature, 'just' and balanced. In other words, I wished the spring water coming down from the mountain was sparkling, when it is not its nature. Instead of drinking abundantly of it and enjoying all its benefits, **I wanted it to become something else,** with other characteristics. And this is, I believe, the mistake I made.

I didn't fully enjoy, in essence, what Cosmos Point represents, but **I wanted to model it to my idea.** As for the tibetan bowl, I advise that **you centre** a few minutes and then **let its action be,** diffused itself. Leave the tea, which you put in hot water, infused so that you can have a beverage which will give you satisfaction.
When you think that its effect grows weaker, start over again. What is interesting is that, the more you use it, the more **you will get a long resonance.** From a few instants at first, you can have a few minutes later…and more.

I - Cosmos Points and Protection

In energetics, we are paying a particular attention to **the protection of the operator.** Since I practice, I meet many practitioners who finish their session **emptied of their energies**.

Schools like Reiki and Quantum Touch are teaching that it doesn't happen with their processes. However, after a day full of sessions, and even practicing *'protection rituals'*, I was done.

I often questioned myself on practioners protection. Beliefs which have been taught to me, were that **we do not use our own energy but the unlimited universal one.** However, it didn't prevent negative returns. The only process I found coherent and actually **non-tiring** is Ho'oponopono. **We work on ourself to change the partner.** By practicing it a few years ago and having the chance to go to Hawaï, I realised that it might be **a real answer.** With the Cosmos Point and the Connection Contact (next chapter), I chose to explain what is happening **from an inside out perspective.**

Not like traditional healers who use THEIR own energies to appease clients…but more that the **connection to the Universe** doesn't go through, as in Reiki type styles, **from an external source,** but from **our internal Universe** which is a small version and with the macrocosm characteristics of the Universe.

We are not anymore in the reception of a force, but we are simultaneously the **transmitter and container** of the energy. As **we do not try to project** or to integrate energies, we avoid receiving and therefore tiring. **The protection** of the operator is **possible with centring on his/her Cosmos Point.** The reason has nothing to do with the energetic. **Trance in which you enter** will centre yourself toward this positive state you can live. This trance allows you to be **more attentive to yourself,** your needs, your instincts. It offers you a **capacity to avoid** negative people or to **not take personally** things that are expressed. By doing so, you are looking for the good, the fair, and there is very little chance that the negative points will be emphasised.

It is important that you remember that **the heart of Cosmos Points is the trance** made available. From this trance, you open possibilities and the only limit is your beliefs.

J – Some leads

In addition to these simple techniques, there are other interesting things that you can do with Cosmos Point.

It is possible to **learn things quicker** even to instinctively understand the functioning of a tool, instrument, practice and to succeed to assimilate things more easily. As we could connect to a **Universe source** (Superconscious) which allows us to remember that we always knew and that we just needed to open the right door to make it work again. It is actually the reason why I named these points, Cosmos Points, this link with our **internal energy which enclose the Universal energy.**

Thanks to this centring, I had patients who gain instantly confidence, make disappear a phobia, fear, anxiety, a thought… A child can succeed to read more easily and fluently while centring. Doors **of possibilities stay open to your ideas.** You just have to keep in mind the functioning of the point to get to these exceptional results.

Chapter 4 : The Connection Contact Touching (CCT)

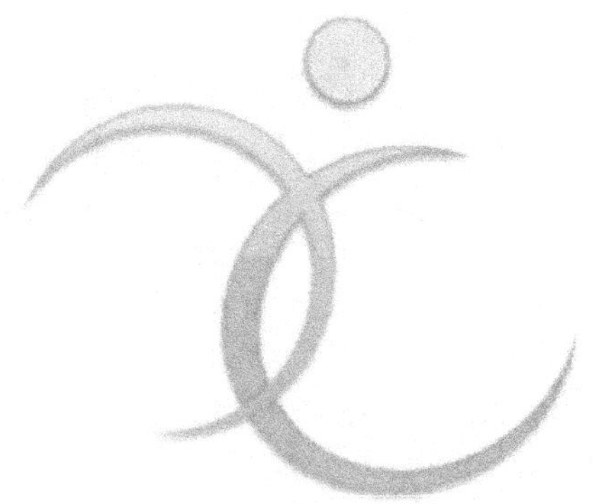

Since I practice energetics, The Connection Contact (CC) is the easiest process I worked with. Even easier than Cosmos Points. I can't, at the moment, give you any rational explanations, I will work on it and indicate to you my thoughts in my next books.

I found this method following works on Cosmos Points. Observing in Martial Arts what these points could do, I remembered a concept I was teaching to my students in Mixt Martial Arts/JiuJitsu class, a prehension art close to Judo. I was then explaining that you just need to touch (connect) a part of the body with the part which was making the effort, so that the **effort diminishes and the resistance multiplies.**

As I did many physical tests with the Cosmos Points, like the resistance to punches, the possibility to multiply the impact of percussions…etc, I made the link between this connection and the cosmos points.

I took back my experiences with a simple principle : when I make a move, **I always keep a hand in contact with my body. Results were almost the same.** Maybe a little less obvious on certain aspects but I found a big part of the results previously obtained. From there, I wondered if **what was making an impact, was also appeasing, calming and helping** others. I started then to test this connection on everyone. As I always do my hypnosis session in touching my clients on the shoulder, I realised that **they were going quicker in deep trances.** By shaking the 'connected' hand, I realised that in an instant, *the breathing and tensions of the person were calming down.* The more I multiplied experiences, the more I realised that **people were quickly appeased**, that their pains were gone or diminished, stress disappeared. *They were all entering trances,* close to the somnanbulant level. By the way, the first time I propose to people who knew well hypnosis, they confirmed with me that sensations were **very similar from entering a trance.** I took back the same principles as for cosmos point. At first, I only was doing a **touch connect to a part of myself,** then I started to put in an intention.

I propose that you make an exercise. It is very easy, the only constraint is **to have a receptive person,** meaning who can feel well changes in his/her body. If you have noone but a cat or a dog, you can try on them aswell. It is actually impressive to see the results on animals.

- Ask your partner how he/she feels on a scale of 1 to 10
- Put your hand on his/her shoulder, stay like this for a few moments
- Ask your partner how he/she feels on a scale of 1 to 10
- Connect your hand to your heart, while keeping the other hand on the shoulders of your partner
- Stay and observe how your partner breathes, tensions in his/her body
- Ask your partner how he/she feels on a scale of 1 to 10
You will see that if his/her eyes are open, the eyes are fixed, it is normal, **he/she entered into a receptive trance** by *internal focus*. Observe what changed and question him/her.
If he/she has closed eyes, you will observe that he/she is most likely to have glazing eyes. It is also a trance.

With this simple way of doing, you are able to have results quite similar to a lot of other energetics processes. Some will say : is it just that ? Yes, it is exactly that, however, we can also amplify the technique. As for Cosmos Points, you can **put in an Intention**. As I thought it was not really 'palpable' to say if the appeasement or the well being was increasing or not, I went back to physical experiences. Admittedly, it is said that **an intention can easily pass time and space.** Maybe you read already the experience of prayer. If we take two groups with the same hurts, that one of them has the support (without knowing it) of a prayer group and the other one not, there is an obvious improvement of the group supported. **It is the power of the intention.**
All this is very interesting on paper, but **how to verify it ?**
I started back tests with punches.

- Punch on a body part of the partner without connection/ without intention
- *'Connected' Punch* with similar returns to Cosmos points
- *'Connected' Punch* and intention

1) <u>Intention of anger</u> : The punch is hurftful but doesn't diffuse
2) <u>Intention of hate</u> : The punch is very precise, like as if the impact would only stay in one place
3) <u>Intention of love</u> : The punch diffuses itself like a 'blast'

After tested a few times, even in boxing, without my partners knowing it, I have seen changes. I am always very careful to not look for the KO, to not create the trauma. However, **with a connection and a love intention,** I without willing, put out of conciousness two partners in 2 weeks. Both have made the same description, the punch has 'spread' over the body. The love notion, as it is given to us in books, whether spiritual or in personal development, is expressed as an **unlimited force, a force which spread.** And as strange as it can look, *to hit someone with 'love' is stronger than to hit with hatred.* Surprising physical observation.
Anyway, I have tested other words, other intentions and **the word love stays the one which 'spread' the most.** I even tested the word in French, Spanish or German, and we still get the same feedback. There is also the word **God** which offer powerful effects. Now, I didn't use all the words of the dictionary, tests are still demanding for the body (we are definately not made to punch ourselves, more to **hug each other with Love**).

Here is the process I put in place for the Connection Contact :
- Put your hand on your heart (or elsewhere)
- Touch your partner
- Think or repeat to yourself the word 'Love'.

Here, you master the process. You are going to be able to do magnetism on almost all pains, physical or moral hurts. I really like this technique and **really want to broadcast it**. I have put all explanations online, on my youtube and shared it with a maximum of people. I think that this method, with this simplicity, *offers to anyone the possibility to bring a better being to others.* Therefore, there is no training or money to spend in order to practice. If after testing this method, you find good results and you are happy about it, I will ask one thing : **share it for free with** everyone who might be interested.
Having been trained in many styles, I found that some processes were not worth the price, Maybe some of you think that **magnetism is a gift.** That it is transmitted generation to generation. I often meet people who have been told that they have a healing gift. Good news, **we all have.** Actually, this belief prevented me entering into the GNOMA (French group of Magnetiser) who gather the 'real' magnetisers. Long story short, I have luckily met three of them whith whom exchanges were great and during which I had to demonstrate my magnetism. In the last meeting, the man who evaluated me, didn't question my competencies, however he didn't appreciate when I said that **magnetism is not a gift**, that everyone has it, that it requires work on it to be able to help.

As I wasn't talking about my 'family line', I became persona non grata. I admit that I was very disappointed, I really thought that I would meet great people in this group.

Let **your kids try to do the Connection Contact.** I had feedback from a mother who taught it to her daughter of 8 years old. This mom, a little bloated, told her condition to her daughter who immediately applied what she had been taught and appeased the discomfort of her mother. As in Cosmos Points, you will observe that **partners enter into trances** very quickly. It happens often that they live things which will **disturb them, flashes, emotions.** It is normal, remember that it is a possibility in any dialogue. Subconscious can offer informations **not rationally understood** by conscious and which will **then express themselves through the body.**

Connection Contact on yourself

We can **work on ourselves** with Connection Contact. Indeed, if there is one thing I appreciated with Reiki, is that the first step which is proposed to learners, is to work for a little while on themselves **before trying on someone else.** It is **an opportunity** to be able to work on yourself when we have pains, anxiety or otherwise.
You already know how to do Cosmos Points. With Connection Contact, it is even easier. After a few 'researches' to optimise the **self-care method,** I found different techniques. I would advise to try and modify them to your convenience.

<u>**1) One hand on your heart, the other one on the painful part**</u>

It is a basic in all magnetism schools. We can put **our hand, where the discomfort is.** It is a way to learn to *'listen to our hands'.* I advise then, to put one hand on the painful part, if it is inaccessible, try on the opposite side of the hurt. For example : For a painful back, put your hand on your chest.

The hand on the hurt **is better flat,** now, if only one finger stays in contact it is perfect aswell, **do not limit yourself into forms.** You just need to keep in mind that *you are connecting.*

The other hand stays close to the heart. When I say 'heart', it is in order to keep **the love symbolic, the 'mantra'which you repeat to yourself.** So, I only talk about a symbol, no obligation.

To sum up :
- One hand on the heart
- One hand on the hurt

To this, you will just need to **add the chosen intention.** I would, again, advise to use 'Love', but you will find what works best for you.

<u>Time :</u>
It is not useful to determine an amount of time, if your pain disappears quickly, stop. If you do not see any changes, no worries, stop and go back to it later on. **5 minutes** is a reasonable amount of time. Of course, you can do more.

What is hapenning ? :

You enter into a trance, **a healing trance,** or at least one of better being. **This trance is open** to receive suggestions, in particular **the word Love**. Moreover, you offer yourself **a contact with your being**. Contact is not valued in our societies. We are afraid to hold, stroke, massage. To give yourself a contact, an attention, seems rare. Self-care is a good way to give yourself this little joy. Also, **we release an energy,** we put then a link between our trance and this intention and this contact. *We open the possibility to integrate :* Love, happiness, well being instead of body hurts. *We replace hurts with a word,* then a vibration.

2) The Prayer Hand

Thinking of the different ways to connect, I had a **mudra phase.** A mudra is a posture that we take with our hands to make things within ourself circulate, for example, to free our breathing, calm down stress… It is a technique Yogis have used for ever. I thought that **contact between the thumb and the index finger** was a way to make us enter a trance. Having done it a lot during Pranayama Yoga, I entered immediately different states when I took different postures with my hands and my fingers. After a few experiences, I realised that the touch *wasn't manifest enough.* As if I was too dissociated, when this technique should allow us to connect. I then, studied another way, the **palm against palm** that we know in prayer and which the Japanese named Gasho.

Following a hurt in the middle of my back, I put in place a Connection Contact with the principle of 'prayer'.

I **connected my hands with a love intention** and in a few minutes, my pain resorbed. It is also possible that praying, meditating a lot in this posture, trance anchored in this position and that automatically *I let' good things' happen.* It opened a reflection about people who heal by faith and prayers. We *connect two parts of ourselves, symbolically, yin (left) with yang (right).* There is then **a spontaneous connection contact. Moreover, faith is the most powerful lever for our spirit.**

This combination of factors offers really significant changes in body and spirit. This method is really **efficient and very discrete,** not like others. Indeed, it is easy to connect your hands…no obligation to make your fingers point to the sky. **The principle palm against palm is perfect.** Put into it an intention and simply listen to your interior.

3) Top of the Skull

This method came to me in Auto Hypnosis. I was in a very deep trance and I asked to my subconscious, in which part of my head was this state. I felt suddenly **the top of my skull 'vibrating'.** It is not the Coronal Chakra, just a little lower.

When I finished my trance, I wanted to test again on myself. And by just laying hands on my head, I went back very quickly into trance. As I know that I am conditioned to go into trance very easily, I started to test on clients during sessions. And I found out that, for the majority of them, just to touch this part of their head **facilitated an open trance.**

To use Connection Contact, just **put your hands on your head and orientate your intention,** towards yourself or the discomfort.
Very easy to apply even during a meeting.

4) Works conclusion on self-care

Works on self-care do not replace doctors or medicine. It allows a *regulation of your own energy.* With a fluid energy, Chinese and Indians teach us that we can avoid excesses and deficiency. *The more we find a balance, the less we get sick.* It even gets more interesting, *it is not that we do not get sick, it is more that we get only very little sickness.* This concept, I discoverd as a teenager in a process called Seitai. It explains mainly that **to never be sick is not a good thing** as the occidental society would like us to believe. Indeed, if our body has symptoms, it is in a way because it frees things. It is a **form of expression for our subconscious,** what we name *somatisation.* You know that our subconscious tries to communicate with our conscious, except that we have a critical factor preventing the full understanding or acceptance of messages. The body is a next step, to make us 'be aware' that **something needs our attention.** Unless we are perfectly good in our communication, it happens that we somatise, sometimes simple things, sometimes more complex illnesses. To come back to Seitai, practitioners think that illness **should not be taken as a problem, but as the expression of the problematic** (we keep the same principle in CT). The goal is to **listen enough to yourself so that symptoms can live their cycle quickly.** Just like having a flu for one day, one evening.

They even go further, explaining that this expression of the body, and by extension I would say subconscious, **is a necessity,** because we then **become more 'sensitive' to our spiritual hurts, and so to our physical hurts.**
It is true that often people who never got sick, when they do, develop big symptoms like cancer or else. Seitai and CT works around the idea that the patient has not been able to hear the small signals. So *the only signal 'understood' became bigger. We are not strong in being deaf to ourselves, we are strong because we are sensitive to ourselves.* Working with self-care, **we regulate** and even if we get sick, **we succeed to reduce the amount of time** of the illness. We are more able to modify things which aren't working, to arrive to a quick and positive conclusion.

By repeating healing trances, we are more in contact with ourselves and we anchor them into our life, which allows us to **integrate strong suggestions for subconscious and body.** The more we work our trances, and so our Connection Contact, the more we **open longterm possibilities** to be more in harmony with ourselves.

Chapter 5 : Cosmos Point and Connection Contact

I have shared two simple ways to propose magnetism to your partners. Cosmos Points allows you **to centre yourself on you** and to transmit an intention. Connection Contact – Touching functions through our **capacity to connect us to ourselves and to enter into contact with our partner.** You can imagine that it is **possible to link them both.** *Everything remains very simple, we are going to combine our centring, our connection and create a contact with an intention towards our partner.*
It is for now, the most elaborate way I have developed. It offers extraordinary opportunities in energetics to help others.
- Centre yourself to your Cosmos Point
- Connect yourself to the part of your body
- Contact your Partner

You now know how to do this.

<u>On what can we use this process ?</u>

We really can use these two processes on everything.

Just remember that **everyone lives things his/her own way.** Even if it can be difficult to accept, everyone has his own rhythm, everyone lives the different therapies in his/her own way, whether they are manual, psychological or energetic.

We are not others, we can't decide for them what is good for them and what is not. In the same way, we can't go faster than them. **We support them** and we are not at all 'healers' in its proper sense. **The only healer is the partner,** who will start **his/her own force to come back to a healthy place**. This potential, all humans have it, it is important to keep that in mind. *We are not doing anything else than to support him/her in his/her own approach.* In Energetics CT, it is primordial to **stay in our just place,** if you already are a therapist, you know this. However, if you enter into personal care, it is important to remember it.

I find that the philosophy of energetic is **a good school for humility.** And very often people, who have practiced, a lot these different processes, are not result dependant. Learning during years that **we only are recipients of an energy** which we propose to others, places us into a very neutral role. It is less the case for *a practitioner who looks for the* 'flaw' in the process partner, which will orientate him/her to a life-saving awareness. *To develop then, the low position is often more difficult with this kind of discipline.* This **energetic wisdom** is a key element of CT. It offers us our just place as a practitioner, helper, supporter and not the **all powerful** technician of a discipline.

Keeping this philosophy, you really can open the domain of applications for these energetic principles. I propose here a **non exhaustive listing** of different aches you can help with. Some concern heavy illnesses, and I want to be clear here, it is **not about healing them,** simply to appease pains, sometimes for hours, sometimes for days :

- Skin Disease
- Burns
- Itching
- Back issues
- Diverse pains
- Sleep
- Weight
- Cigarettes
- Cancer
- Multiple Sclerosis
- Anxiety
- Stress
- Depression
...

At the start of my practicing in energetic, I really tried it out on everyone, whatever issues, physical or psychological.
I discovered surprising things. Keep in mind that *if there are no positive effects…there will be no negatives aswell.*

Chapter 6 : Distant Healing

If there is a difficult thing to admit in our actual world, it is the notion of **a distant energetic transfer.**

The idea of entering into trances when we receive an energetic session is more and more accepted. In the same way you will find that the idea, of the partner **entering into trances via internal focusing,** provoking a form of self-suggestion of better being, is also accepted. However, the idea that, without any contact, someone can work on someone else, with physical and psychic results, seems completely unlikely. **I understand,** and I will not try to make you change your mind. I will just simply expose different things. Firstly, here is how I started to experiment this idea. Frankly, **I didn't believe in it at all.** Keeping in mind the idea that **energy and intention have no limit or constraint,** I sent energies to people I knew weren't doing well. Without asking, without them knowing it, I was imagining that my energy passed to them. My hands were empty while **'perceiving' my partner under them.**

For example :

- An internal focus
- Open a capacity to **Act as If,** which put me into trance
- In Trance, I connect myself to Supraconscious (also known as Morphogenetic field)
- 'Diffuse' into it an intention or a suggestion

The intention can be a **facet of this energy** of life that we treat in energetic styles.

Effects of this 'trying' sessions were interesting, however, automatically **they build a doubt,** the need to know if the work influences really the better being.

The second way was to complete the partners session with a remote session. With the same process. With years, the discovery of concepts such as Ho'oponopono, and a better comprehension of the mirror effect, I really did stick to a few concepts. Especially the one which developed the idea that **sick people are a part of us.** Our goal being to 'clean' the ache within us. I went from a **quite ritualised process** to enter trance, to a quick connection capacity into **an open magnetism trance.** I completed then my sessions during my free time, meaning walking, watching a movie, with friends. Here is how I use it still :

- Centre myself on the person. At first I kept an image but then just a word representing the person was enough.
- Focus on his/her issue
- Repeat to myself simply a kind of mantra as 'I welcome and clean this sickness in me'.

Thanks to this, I was able to make a 'double impact'. I **work on the other one while working on me.** It is a **balance of giving to the other and giving to oneself.** For a while, friends and partners were texting me when pain was taking them. I was then putting in place the previous process. After a few minutes or hours, it happened that I received positive feedbacks from them. Here again, it can be explained with the trance I was into and **the effect of resonance from me to others.** For example, if you feel good and that your friends lack energy, it is easy to diffuse your dynamic to the group.

That is what I call a **resonance effect.** Your well being, your vitality and your positive attitude boost the ones around you. You can try it, it is verifiable. With the Mantra of Ho'oponopono process, you can have excellent results. Let me remind you :'**I am sorry, Forgive me, Thank you, I love you'.** Keep in mind this sentence or at least its concept, we are going to come back to it.

Apart from the principle of trance and resonance. There is also a particular posture for the recipient : **the awaiting** and the **internal focusing.** These two elements allow you, as you know, to go into trance.

For example, the process could be :
- Request to receive energetic
- **Strong focus on internal sensations** in the body
- **Awaiting for changes.** This phase opens even more trance and possible potentials.
- **Auto-Suggestions** are possible on the desire to feel better and to feel something.

Most of remote sessions will gather these elements :
1) Pratitioner into **Trance** and in an **Intention posture**
2) Partner in **Trance** and in **awaiting of change posture**

Apart from trance, intention offers a possibility to transmit positive elements, even **palpable for the recipient.**

<u>**How Energetics CT works in remote sessions ?**</u>

We studied two different tools : Cosmos Points and Connection Contact – Touching. We validated the capacity of the operator of these techniques to enter into trances. Now, we are going to stay on the most simplest approach. In my opinion, a process should always be easy, so that a large number of people can master the technique. Let's take the first way of doing, Cosmos Points. You are, again, going to be able to work on **Advanced Centring.**

<u>***Cosmos Point and remote work***</u>

Technique 1 :

1) Centre yourself on your Cosmos Point
2) Contact with your harmony Trance
3) Send thought of the person towards your Cosmos Point. Act as if you were thinking with your cosmos point.
4) Put his/her image in the same harmonious state you are living in
5) Once you are fully appeased and that the image is more 'healthy', stop.

It will take you **around 3 minutes.**
The key point is really to *focus your thought on the point and to imagine the person better and better.* It allows you to **stay on yourself** and the state that is the most **positive for yourself.** You are never either *'getting out' of yourself, nor receiving from the outside any forces.* You are careful to yourself and so to the person in demand.

Technique 2 :

1) Centre yourself on your Cosmos Point
2) Contact with your harmony Trance
3) Look in your Cosmos Point the part of yourself which suffers as your partner
4) Welcome the hurt
5) Then welcome your aptitude to be perfectly healthy

We are in the **notion to welcome all things in life.**
It doesn't mean that we are accepting hurts and sicknesses, **but we welcome their existence.** *We accept then, the other one (our partner) as a part of ourselves.* Once this step is completed, **we welcome our own capacity to be fully healthy** and full of energy, and so that our partner, who is part of us, is too. This technique may seem a little bit complex on paper, but really isn't. Quite the opposite, **it is really simple.** In a few minutes only, we can have important effects.
You can observe that in the two basic techniques, we remain **very linked to ourselves.** Above all, an important element is **to not lose yourself in the other one or any outside element**. You notice, if you are into remote magnetism, that when you are using Cosmos Point, it is possible **that you lose your sensitivity in your hands.** I realised in my case, and before I had effervescent hands while doing direct or remote magnetism, that with Energetics CT tools, I can even have **my hands completely cold.** So, no worries if you do not experience exactly how methods are described.

I propose to you a set of tools and ways to apply them, **but the most important is to listen to yourself.** In trances, we are able to do incredible things. We are open to ourself and connected to the other one so *our spontaneity, without form, will be the best teacher.*

Connection Contact and remote work

In my opinion, Connection Contact requests less work than Cosmos Point. You just have to touch a part of your body. For the remote work, it is easy to connect with yourself…it is more delicate to operate the contact as your partner is not right in front of you.

There are two applications :
- The first one is quite old school. Your hand remains palm up or down, as if you were touching the person, either on the hurt or the shoulder.
- The second is to use **the prayer hand posture.** In this case, just imagine that you write, photograph or hold the partner in your hands. I imagine **simply first names, as to enter in contact.** It is a known method for…remote clairvoyance…when I say that all disciplines use the same path.

You just have to choose one of the two postures and you can start to work.

Technique 1 : Basic

- Contact and connect yourself to your partner

- Build an intention of better being for the person treated.
- The most important is to stay connected.
- After a few minutes, stop.

I can imagine that it is hard to believe that it is all that needs to be done. **I invite you not only to believe but to experiment and observe.** Before writing this part of the book, I wanted to verify with a number of experiences what I propose to you today. To do so, I proposed via the website www.partage-energetique.jimdo.com small sessions to boost the energetic. I have been overwhelmed by demands, which has been a great surprise. I was then able to work on different issues with the tools I propose to you now. This basic technique allowed people who were suffering from diverse causes such as back pain, recurrent migraines, insomnia, lack of energy…etc, to feel better. I insist on the **feel better,** I consider that we are not healing anyone, we *just offer an additional way for the body to find back its well being.*

There is a second method which uses the welcoming concept other than Cosmos Point, but with **more Ho'oponopono semantic.**

<u>***Technique 2 : Cleansing of the being***</u>

Step 1

- Contact and connect yourself to your partner
- Start to look for the part which is problematic. For example if your partner has migraine, focus on your head.
- Repeat a first mantra such as :
    - I ask forgiveness for these aches I give myself to my head
    - I authorise my forgiveness to hurt my head.
    - I ask forgiveness for the hurt which resonates in my head.

This first part takes **2 or 3 minutes,** you need to really connect with your request. It is not only the notion 'to be sorry'. Having this mantra tested in many different ways, it appears that **we are all the time sorry in our society.** Conclusion : even **our subconscious doesn't put any energy in it. Looking for forgiveness** is a centring moment extremely important in our quest of better being for our partner. **You can create the mantra you want.** I often have a starting mantra which **changes** after a few minutes of use without me being 'conscious'of it. For example, I will go from : « I ask forgiveness to myself for the ache I have » to « I ask forgiveness for the lack of attention I give to myself ». This progression is positive, in the sense that in Connection Contact, we are into trance and so in direct exchange with **the subconscious which supports us completely in the approach we put in place.**

Step 2

- Repeat a 2nd mantra such as :
  - I ask forgiveness to myself for the hurt I caused to my head.
  - I forgive that I haven't welcomed this ache
  - I forgive myself for taking so long before loving me

This second mantra reflects the 'Forgive me' of Ho'oponopono. Here again, it is important to **not repeat without intention**. I know that in our tradition it is taught that it is enough to repeat the mantra to cleanse yourself. I did it myself for a long time before discovering the famous **Joseph Murphy.** I was spending all my time repeating mantras, for hours, days and even months. Working in hypnosis, I realised that I was able to improve the benefits of mantras if I **associated an emotion to them** more. This is the reason why I'd rather propose to you a **lever to your trance,** to use an emotion and let your subconscious bring you what it desires to transmit through your work.

Step 3

- Repeat these last mantras : **Thanks, and I welcome the unconditional love.**

Learning to **be full of gratitude and love with yourself** is a sensation that we need to feel, even for only a few moments. Indeed, it happens often that we are not able to **love ourself to our true value** and that we spend our time devaluing ourselves. To open ourselves, **even for a few minutes, to respect and love** towards ourselves offers us extraordinary possibilities.

To put this in place within you, you are going to spend **around 10 to 15 minutes.** It is a bit longer than the other methods. The work gives great results and comes from a vision, a belief that **we are all linked one to another.** It proposes a philosophy, *if we want to change this around, we need to change things within us.*

These two techniques can of course, if you want, **be helped with a centring in Cosmos Point.** There are then a few variations. You can test this.

To conclude, I really want you to keep in mind, that this particular aspect of energetics, is **a little plus to the different methods you will propose to your partners.** It offers results, more or less obvious. I will advise that you **always complete them with face to face sessions.** Even if the recipient partners are into trance and that we are too, to share this with a physical presence is always **in full, more sincere, more true.** It is a bit like giving…you can always give money towards hunger…it will never be like going and feeding someone yourself. In our encounter, we offer a little bit of our heart.

Chapter 7 : Partners perception

Like in many disciplines you will propose, there is a big chance that your partners have **strong expectations.**

As I explain in CT or hypnosis, *expectation can be your worst enemy for any change.* It has to be **a part of the process,** however, it can't **be excessive.** Indeed, all techniques, and especially the ones looking a bit like magic **develop excess.** Most of the time, there are two types of partners who will go and see an 'energetician' or a 'magnetiser'. Those who are themselves in this dynamic, they know it and have a good image of it because someone they know has tested it. And those who have tested everything else, **they have no more hope** and wait for a **miracle** through what the practitioner will propose.

I advise that **you take some time to redefine** expectations and beliefs. You can explain to them that you are simply **going to work on their own capacities of healing. Explain your role** and pay extra attention to remove anything mystical in their vision of a magnetiser. I know that some people, in hypnosis as in all other disciplines, like to keep **'an absolute power' facet.** It is a double edged sword. Indeed, during trance, the partner can **develop faith in you or in your 'force'.** This will considerably help the process of the well being. However, It can also become such **an expectation to live something out of the ordinary,** that if he/she doesn't live up to the idea he/she has, and even if all went well, *it might be that he/she stays on his/her deception and even maybe sabotage himself/herself with negative suggestions.* Demystifying, **you offer the just place to your action.**

You also offer to your partner the possibility to be **responsible for his/her session.** He/she becomes entirely part of the process. There are different ways, therefore, for the partner to react. *As operator, you do not need to have any expectations on the perception of your partners.* Let them live things in their own way. Here are some perceptions your partners can have :

- Pins and needles
- Warmth
- Cold
- Pressure
- Dizziness
- Feeling nauseous
- Laughter
- Cries
- Shivers
- Awakening pains
- Moving pains
- Discomfort variations : high then low, or opposite
- Hallucinations
- Euphoria
- Complete relaxation
- Tension
- Cardiac rhythm change
- Breathlessness
- Anxiety
- Oppression
- Fear
- …

There can be others, these ones are the most '*common*'.

Pay attention to the reactions of your partners. This aspect is part of your work. I always say that energetic can't hurt. And it is true but not necessarily the way we think. Indeed, a few years ago when I was studying in some schools, I used to think that **my sessions would be gentle.** I was though warning that, during a **21 days cycle,** some variations could happen. This is by the way advise that I give you, explain that **in three weeks, things can vary** in the life of the partner. However, I was not expecting that even from session to session, **there would be so much happening.** Indeed, using styles you already know or Energetics CT tools, you will discover that during session, things change. It happens often that a person who comes for a pain see **his/her pain explode during a few minutes during the session.** Again, I remind you to ask your partner to **give a scale** from 1 to 10 of his/her pain so that you can follow the perception of your partner. When someone has a persistent pain of 5 and after a few minutes **the pain explodes to 10** and moves itself, **stay calm** and keep going. Your sessions can **last 45 minutes.** Though with experience, I can testify that **time is not at all a guarantee of quality.**

The energy and the subconscious take **all information and changes in the instant.** A thought is immediate, a suggestion is directly understood without any effort. *Feedbacks are also immediate.* For example, think of the taste of ginger bread. Some will smile at this thought as they like it, some others will be disgusted, and some will even have memories coming to them.

This idea travelled in half a second and your subconscious, **in an instant, offered you a return :** an emotion, a taste, a memory or otherwise. It is the same thing during sessions, and this is why sometimes in 3 minutes, your partner could not feel his/her pain which will never come back. So, if it is not the case. If the pain increases, or fears, or anxiety, simply carry on with your work **until appeasement.** Remember that work in energetics, as I see it, open trances. I remind you again, it is a communication between conscious and subconscious without barrier. When you transfer your intention, energy, you give the possibility to your partner to let his/her subconscious and body express themselves fully. However, they have been **muzzled for years, of their words and hurts.** As you open the communication, their expression can be shaking. This is why, a **certain amount of time for assimilation, going deeper, during the 21 days.** Schemes which have been destructured and changed, need to **find their new place** in the body, spirit of the operator and then stabilised. **Always warn beforehand** that sessions can be lively and disturbing.

When I was in my testing phase, and that I was doubting a lot about magnetism, I tried many ways. At this time, I really wanted to discover if energetic had a full efficiency without the intervention of psyche. I admit now that **both are necessary.** I had a period where I received my partners and, like **orthodox psychologists,** I wouldn't say a word, not even to the partner. The partner would arrive, sit down, I was doing my session, he/she payed and then went away. It wasn't a very warm environment. Of course, it did help me to gather feedbacks, to know two things : *can we help without knowing the ache ?*

Does the partner feel something after the session ? It appears that for most cases, both answers were positive. We can, without knowing what the person is suffering from, appease him/her. And, there is a change/movement after the session. However, as I wasn't warning partners, some would call me after in a panic at any time of the day or night. I thought it was better to not say anything on the possible effects in post-session, **to not suggest anything.** Partners are really sensitive to our suggestions either physical or psychic at the end of a session. However as, **without warning,** clients still live post-session effects, I **decided to warn them**.

We shouldn't dream of a unique session. It is often the case of many magnetisers, and also a nice place for our ego to tell ourselves…*in one session, partners have been cured of recurrent aches.* I really like the idea of a school I practiced (I can't remember if it is Reiki or mirror body). It proposes 4 sessions :
- 1st Session : Discovery of the body and spirit of energies and practitioner
- 2nd and 3rd Session : Deep work on the issue and harmonising changes
- 4th Session : Conclusion

I had a period where I was only working like this. Then I moved to 3 sessions which seemed more just. Warn your partner that **you will have to see each other a few times** and that remote sessions are not included in the set of sessions.

Conclusion

This first volume about Energetics CT presented to you the main techniques I put in place through the discovery of Cosmos Points and Connection Contact.

These tools are not better than others. Key ideas are **simplicity and centring on oneself.** To not look for an external link but more to **find this unlimited internal force within us.** It may be that some explanations seem weird, especially if you come from the magnetism world. The notion of trance is very specific and maybe, it won't resonate with your beliefs and experiences. It doesn't matter, it is more **a possible explanation than an absolute truth. Techniques work whether we adhere or not to the trance principle.** Take your time to experiment and add to them methods you already use. To all, I sincerely advise you to take a moment to study your type of personality through Enneagram types. This quest is worth it.

Cosmos points will really **open doors to a better being.** There is a progression in the way to perceive your being and life. I will certainly write other books, more complete on facets of Cosmos Points and their **daily use.** Please, note that this discovery is recent, so feel free to share your feedback to me.

Connection Contact – Touching is the technique I **would like the most to broadcast**. It is so simple, so quick to learn and teach, that I think it should be shared and not sold. This method doesn't require training, meditations, beliefs, symbols or initiations. So please, if you are satisfied by the results, **share it freely.** You can also send me your feedback and testimony.

The cleansing work will also be a real addition into your lives. If you are open to it, come and check what the Ho'oponopono proposes. What I propose here is my vision and most of all my return on experiences. *The more we accept ourselves, love ourselves, the more the world around us grows, changes and evolves.* Our perceptions grow and we are not stuck into dark filters anymore.
Energetics CT is **not a frozen concept,** I will evolve, grow, meet people and learn…also my perceptions, beliefs and comprehension will change.

Take from this book and from all my books, only **what is good and just for you.** Take what resonates and makes you vibrate. Create your own way to perceive and to live CT when you practice it. **Do not freeze yourself into forms.** I had to put words on paper, these words are meant to evolve. It is an exploration. It is not because you are not going to say or do what I wrote here that you won't do any extraordinary things. Stay more focused on yourself and your partner than what a book, a video teaches.

You can contact me directly by mail : hype.ose@gmail.com

Pank, Le Chesnay (Dec-2013)

Who is Christophe Pank ?

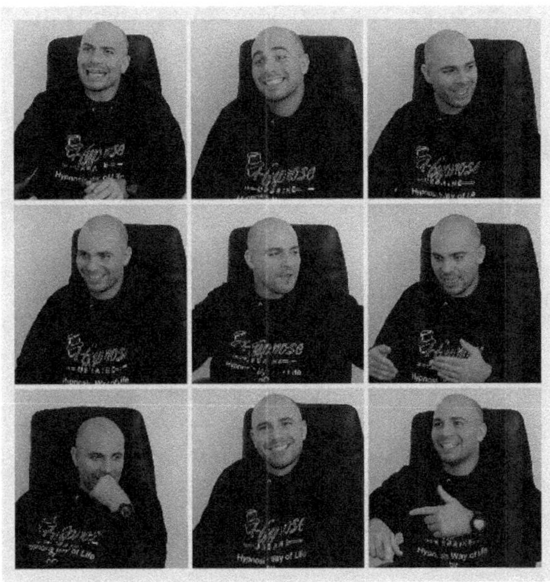

I am French and live in Paris. I have worked in hypnosis, NPL, personal development and energetic healing for more than a decade. Everyday, I share my experience and knowledge. To optimise my work, I created HnO (Hype-N-Ose) Hypnose in 2010. As psycho-practitioner, I can help people to learn about themselves, to increase their knowledge.

I am now sharing my ideas in essays, videos and audios.
The more you open your mind to different ways of
thinking, the more you develop your capacity to become
who you really are.

Take the time to watch my english Youtube Channel :
hnohypnosis and my website : www.hnohypnosis.com